I0757387

Bryan Dorsey, M.D

OUTSMART BLOOD SUGAR

A no-bullshit Guide to Preventing Disease, Losing Weight and Living Healthier

Copyright © 2023 Dr. Bryan Dorsey, M.D

All Right Reserved

Cover Designed By: Smith Henry

Edited By: Janet Smart

The Scanning, uploading and distribution of this book without permission is a theft of the author's intellectual property if you would like permission to use material from the book (other than for review purposes).

Table of Contents

This page was left blank intentionally

Preface

Picture this: **you're in your mid-thirties, feeling healthy and energetic, and enjoying life with your family and friends**. You've always been relatively active and eat a balanced diet, so you never worry about your health. But one day, you start to feel more tired than usual. You're thirsty all the time, and you're losing weight, despite not changing anything in your lifestyle.

You go to the doctor, hoping for a quick fix, but what you hear changes everything. You have high blood sugar, so you're at risk for developing diabetes. You feel a sense of shock and disbelief. How could this happen? You've never thought about blood sugar before. You don't even know what it is.

That was my wake-up call, leading me to write this book.

As a health and wellness coach, I've seen countless clients struggle with blood sugar issues, from prediabetes to type 2 diabetes. Many of them come to me feeling overwhelmed and confused, with little understanding of how their blood sugar affects their health. And I get it – the science behind blood sugar regulation can be complicated, and there's a lot of conflicting information.

But here's the thing: blood sugar isn't just a number on a lab report. It's a key player in your overall health and well-being. And the good news is that there are simple, practical steps you can take to manage your blood sugar and improve your health.

That's why I wrote this **no-bullshit guide to outsmart blood sugar**. This book isn't about quick fixes or magic pills. It's about giving you the knowledge and tools to control your blood sugar and live your best life.

In these pages, you'll learn:

- The science behind blood sugar and how it affects your health

- The common misconceptions about blood sugar and weight loss
- The principles of the blood sugar solution and how to put them into practice
- How to eat for blood sugar health, including a detailed guide to the best foods for regulating blood sugar
- The role of exercise, stress management, supplements, and medications in blood sugar control
- How to prevent complications of high blood sugar and manage existing conditions

But more than that, you'll learn to take ownership of your health and make lasting lifestyle changes to support your blood sugar and overall well-being. You'll discover that managing your blood sugar isn't about deprivation or strict rules – it's about finding a way of eating and living that works for you.

I won't sugarcoat it (pun intended) – this journey won't be easy. It will require commitment, patience, and a willingness to make changes. But I promise you; it will be worth it. By taking charge of your blood sugar health, you'll not only prevent disease and lose weight but also gain energy, vitality, and a renewed sense of purpose.

So, are you ready to outsmart blood sugar?

If so, let's get started.

Using the Book, the Right Way

Congratulations, you've taken the first step towards outsmarting blood sugar by picking up this book! But reading a book is one thing, and putting the knowledge into practice is another. That's why I want to talk about how to use this book effectively and get the most out of it.

First, it's essential to understand that this book is not a quick fix or a magic pill. It's a comprehensive guide to managing blood sugar and improving overall health. That means implementing the strategies and principles outlined in these pages will take time and effort.

But don't worry; you don't have to do it all simultaneously. Trying to make fewer changes at once can be overwhelming and unsustainable. Instead, I recommend taking a gradual approach and implementing one or two changes at a time. This will allow you to focus on making those changes a habit before moving on to the next.

Another essential thing to remember is that everyone's journey to blood sugar health will be different. The advice and strategies in this book are based on the latest scientific research, but ultimately, you'll need to experiment and find what works best for you. That means being open to trying new things, listening to your body, and adjusting as needed.

So, how can you use this book to outsmart blood sugar effectively? Here are a few tips:

Read the entire book before making any significant changes.

While it can be tempting to jump right into the "how-to" sections of the book, I recommend starting with the introduction and background information. This will give you a solid foundation for understanding blood sugar and its impact on your health. Then, as you read through the rest of the book, take notes and highlight sections that resonate with you.

Set realistic goals.

As I mentioned, making too many changes at once can be overwhelming and unsustainable. Instead, focus on setting one or two realistic goals at a time. For example, start by cutting back on sugary drinks or adding a daily 10-minute walk to your routine. Once those changes become habits, you can add in more.

Track your progress.

Keeping track of your progress can help you stay motivated and see how far you've come. This might mean keeping a food journal, tracking your blood sugar levels, or noting how you feel each day. Use whatever method works best for you.

Feel free to ask for help.

Changing your habits and lifestyle can be challenging, and asking for help is okay. Whether talking to a friend, joining a support group, or working with a health coach, feel free to seek support and guidance.

Remember to be kind to yourself.

This journey will be challenging, and you might experience setbacks. Remember to be kind to yourself and give yourself grace. Every small step you take towards better blood sugar health is a step in the right direction.

In conclusion, using this book effectively is all about taking a gradual, personalized approach and being open to experimentation and adjustment. By following the strategies outlined in these pages, you'll be on your way to outsmarting blood sugar and living your healthiest life.

About the Author

Bryan Dorsey, M.D., is a renowned author and expert in health and wellness. He has authored several books, including "Outsmart Aging," "Outsmart Fat Fast," and "Outsmart Fat Fast Kitchen." His latest book, "Outsmart Blood Sugar," is a comprehensive guide to managing blood sugar levels and improving overall health.

Dr. Dorsey was born and raised in the United States and has been passionate about health and wellness from a young age. He pursued his undergraduate studies in biology and completed his medical degree at a prestigious university. Dr. Dorsey has over 30 years of experience in medicine and has worked with thousands of patients to help them achieve optimal health.

Throughout his career, Dr. Dorsey has been dedicated to educating people about the importance of preventive healthcare. He believes that by taking a proactive approach to health, we can prevent many chronic diseases and live happier, more fulfilling lives. That's why he wrote "Outsmart Blood Sugar" - to empower people with the knowledge and tools they need to take control of their health.

In addition to his work as an author, Dr. Dorsey is also a sought-after speaker and consultant. He has been featured on numerous media outlets and has spoken at conferences and events worldwide. Dr. Dorsey is known for his engaging and approachable style, making complex health concepts accessible to everyone.

Outside work, Dr. Dorsey is an avid traveler who enjoys exploring new cultures and cuisines. He also enjoys spending time with his family and staying active through outdoor activities like hiking and biking.

In conclusion, Dr. Bryan Dorsey is a highly respected author and expert in health and wellness. With over 30 years of experience and a passion for preventive healthcare, he is dedicated to empowering people with the knowledge and tools they need to achieve optimal health. "Outsmart Blood Sugar" is the latest example of his commitment to helping people live their healthiest lives.

Introduction

Sugar in the Blood: The Importance You Can't Ignore!

Blood sugar, or blood glucose, is the primary energy source for the body's cells. It's an essential component of our bodies, allowing us to perform daily activities, maintain brain function, and fuel our muscles during exercise. Despite its importance, many people need help understanding blood sugar and its importance to our health.

This book will look closely at blood sugar, including what it is, how it works, and why it's so important.

What is Blood Sugar?

Blood sugar is a type of sugar that's carried in the bloodstream. It comes from food, specifically carbohydrates like bread, rice, pasta, and fruits. When we eat these foods, our digestive system breaks down the carbohydrates into glucose, which is absorbed into the bloodstream.

Once in the bloodstream, glucose is transported to the body's cells, where it's used as fuel. Insulin, a hormone produced by the pancreas, helps transport glucose from the bloodstream into the cells.

If there's too much glucose in the bloodstream and the body can't use it all, the excess is stored in the liver and muscles as glycogen. When the body needs energy, it can break down glycogen to release glucose into the bloodstream.

How Does Blood Sugar Work?

The body is designed to regulate blood sugar levels to maintain a steady energy supply to the cells. Our blood sugar levels rise when we eat, triggering insulin release from the pancreas. Insulin helps move glucose from the bloodstream into the cells, where it's used for energy.

If blood sugar levels drop too low, the pancreas releases another hormone called glucagon. Glucagon signals the liver to break down glycogen and release glucose into the bloodstream, raising blood sugar levels.

Why is Blood Sugar Important?

- Maintaining stable blood sugar levels is essential for overall health and well-being. When blood sugar levels are too high or too low, it can lead to various health problems.

- High blood sugar, also known as hyperglycemia, can cause damage to blood vessels and nerves over time, leading to complications like heart disease, stroke, kidney disease, and nerve damage.

- Low blood sugar, also known as hypoglycemia, can cause symptoms like shakiness, confusion, dizziness, and in severe cases, unconsciousness.

In addition to these short-term and long-term complications, unstable blood sugar levels can make it harder to manage weight and impact mood and energy levels.

TIPS FOR MAINTAINING HEALTHY BLOOD SUGAR LEVELS

There are several steps you can take to maintain healthy blood sugar levels:

Eat a balanced diet: Include plenty of fiber-rich fruits and vegetables, whole grains, lean protein, and healthy fats.

Watch your portion sizes: Overeating can lead to high blood sugar levels.

Stay active: Regular exercise can help regulate blood sugar levels and improve insulin sensitivity.

Manage stress: High stress levels can raise blood sugar levels, so finding ways to manage stress is essential.

Get enough sleep: Lack of sleep can disrupt hormones that regulate blood sugar levels, so getting adequate sleep is crucial.

Blood sugar is a critical component of our bodies, allowing us to perform daily activities and maintain overall health and well-being. By understanding what blood sugar is, how it works, and why it's so important, we can maintain healthy blood sugar levels and prevent the complications associated with high or low blood sugar.

This page was left blank intentionally

Sugar Shock: The Hidden Link to Chronic Diseases

When we think of sugar, we may only consider its immediate effects on our energy levels and mood. However, the link between blood sugar and chronic diseases is a topic that deserves our attention. High blood sugar levels, over time, can contribute to the developing of a range of chronic diseases.

To understand why this is the case, it's essential to understand what happens to our bodies when we consume sugar. When we eat carbohydrates, such as bread or pasta, our body breaks them down into glucose, which is then transported to our cells for energy. Insulin, a hormone produced by the pancreas, regulates our blood sugar levels by signaling to our cells to absorb glucose from the bloodstream.

When we consume too much sugar, however, our bodies can become resistant to insulin, meaning that our cells don't respond as well as they should. This leads to high glucose levels in the bloodstream, which can cause damage to various organs and tissues throughout the body. Over time, this can contribute to the development of chronic diseases.

One of the most well-known chronic diseases associated with high blood sugar is diabetes. In type 2 diabetes, the body becomes resistant to insulin, and the pancreas can't produce enough to keep up with demand. This results in chronically elevated blood sugar levels, which can cause damage to the nerves, kidneys, eyes, and cardiovascular system over time.

But diabetes is not the only chronic disease linked to high blood sugar levels. Research has shown that elevated blood sugar can also contribute to the development of heart disease, stroke, dementia, and certain types of cancer. One study found that people with high blood sugar levels had a 29% higher risk of developing heart disease than those with lower levels.

The link between blood sugar and chronic diseases is complex, and several factors can contribute to it. For example, excess sugar consumption can lead to inflammation throughout the body, contributing to the development of chronic diseases. Additionally, high blood sugar can lead to the production of advanced glycation end products (AGEs), compounds that can damage proteins in the body and contribute to the development of chronic diseases.

So, what can we do to reduce our risk of chronic diseases related to blood sugar? The most important thing is maintaining healthy blood sugar levels by consuming a balanced diet that is low in added sugars and rich in whole, nutrient-dense foods. Regular exercise and maintaining a healthy weight can also help to improve insulin sensitivity and reduce the risk of chronic diseases.

The link between blood sugar and chronic diseases is a complex and vital topic. By understanding how high blood sugar can contribute to developing these diseases, we can take steps to protect our health and reduce our risk. A balanced diet, regular exercise, and maintaining a healthy weight are all critical components of a healthy lifestyle that can help to keep our blood sugar levels in check and reduce our risk of chronic diseases.

This page was left blank intentionally

Misconceptions about blood sugar and diabetes

Diabetes is a condition that affects millions of people worldwide, and there are many misconceptions surrounding blood sugar and diabetes that can be confusing and even harmful. This book will explore some of the most common misconceptions about blood sugar and diabetes and provide clear and accurate information to help you better understand these conditions.

Misconception #1: Diabetes is caused by overeating sugar

One of the most common misconceptions about diabetes is that it is caused by overeating sugar. While consuming excess sugar can contribute to developing type 2 diabetes, it is not the sole cause. Genetics and lifestyle factors such as obesity and physical inactivity are major risk factors for type 2 diabetes.

Misconception #2: Only overweight or obese people can develop diabetes

While being overweight or obese is a significant risk factor for type 2 diabetes, it is not the only factor. Thin people can also develop diabetes, and there are many cases where people who are overweight or obese do not set the condition.

Misconception #3: Diabetes only affects older people

While it is true that the risk of developing diabetes increases with age, it can also affect people of all ages, including children. The number of young people diagnosed with type 2 diabetes is increasing due to the rise in childhood obesity.

Misconception #4: Diabetes is not a severe condition

Diabetes is a painful condition that can lead to various complications, such as heart disease, kidney disease, nerve damage, and vision problems. It is essential to manage diabetes through lifestyle changes and medication to reduce the risk of these complications.

Misconception #5: People with diabetes cannot eat sugar or carbohydrates

While people with diabetes need to manage their carbohydrate and sugar intake to control their blood sugar levels, it is unnecessary to avoid these foods altogether. A balanced and healthy diet that includes whole, nutrient-dense foods and moderate amounts of carbohydrates and sugar can be incorporated into a diabetes management plan.

Misconception #6: Diabetes can be cured

While diabetes cannot be cured, it can be managed through lifestyle changes and medication. Type 2 diabetes can often be managed through weight loss, physical activity, and healthy eating habits. Type 1 diabetes, on the other hand, requires insulin therapy for life.

Misconception #7: You can tell if someone has diabetes just by looking at them

Diabetes is an invisible condition, meaning that you cannot tell if someone has diabetes just by looking at them. It is essential to be aware of the signs and symptoms of diabetes, such as increased thirst, frequent urination, and blurred vision, and to seek medical attention if you experience these symptoms.

In conclusion, many misconceptions about blood sugar and diabetes can be harmful and confusing. By understanding the facts about these conditions, we can better manage our health and reduce our risk of developing complications. Suppose you are concerned about your blood sugar levels or have been diagnosed with diabetes. In that case, working closely with your healthcare provider to develop a personalized management plan that meets your individual needs is essential.

Know Your Numbers: Monitoring Blood Sugar Levels Made Easy

Maintaining healthy blood sugar levels is crucial for overall health and well-being. The first step towards achieving this is to regularly measure and monitor your blood sugar levels. In this book, we'll discuss the different ways to measure and monitor blood sugar levels.

A blood glucose test is the most common way to measure blood sugar levels. This test involves pricking your finger and placing a drop of blood on a test strip, which is then inserted into a glucose meter. The meter measures the glucose level in your blood and provides a reading within a few seconds.

There are different types of blood glucose tests, including fasting plasma glucose (FPG) test, oral glucose tolerance test (OGTT), and hemoglobin A1C (HbA1c) test. The FPG test requires you to fast for at least eight hours before the test, while the OGTT involves drinking a sugary solution and having your blood sugar levels checked at regular intervals. The HbA1c test measures the average blood sugar levels over the past three months.

Continuous glucose monitoring (CGM) is another way to monitor blood sugar levels. This involves wearing a small sensor on your skin that continuously measures your glucose levels and sends the data to a receiver or smartphone app. CGM is particularly helpful for people with diabetes who must monitor their blood sugar levels frequently.

In addition to blood glucose tests and CGM, there are other ways to monitor blood sugar levels. For instance, some people use urine test strips to measure their blood sugar levels. However, urine test strips are less accurate than blood glucose tests or CGM and are not recommended for regular monitoring.

Monitoring blood sugar levels regularly is essential to identify any fluctuations or changes. Fluctuations in blood sugar levels can lead to various health issues, including diabetes, heart disease, and stroke.

To monitor blood sugar levels effectively, you should log your readings. This can help you identify patterns and adjust your diet, exercise, and medication. You can also share your log with your healthcare provider to help them develop an appropriate treatment plan for you.

This page was left blank intentionally

The Truth About Carbohydrates

Carbs & Blood Sugar: How They Work Together

Carbohydrates are an essential component of our diet, providing energy to fuel our daily activities. However, when it comes to blood sugar regulation, the type and amount of carbohydrates we consume can significantly impact our health.

Carbohydrates are broken down into glucose during digestion, which is then released into the bloodstream. In response, the pancreas releases insulin, a hormone that helps transport glucose from the bloodstream into our cells, which can be used for energy.

Carbohydrates can be divided into two categories: simple and complex. Simple carbohydrates, also known as sugars, are easily and quickly digested, rapidly increasing blood glucose levels. This can result in a spike in insulin levels, causing a quick drop in blood glucose levels, leaving us tired and hungry again soon after eating.

Examples of foods high in simple carbohydrates include candy, soft drinks, fruit juice, and processed snacks. Consuming too much of these types of foods can lead to weight gain and an increased risk of developing type 2 diabetes.

On the other hand, complex carbohydrates take longer to digest, leading to a slower and more sustained release of glucose into the bloodstream. This results in a more gradual increase in blood glucose levels, which can help to maintain energy levels and prevent cravings for high-sugar foods.

Examples of foods high in complex carbohydrates include whole grains, fruits, vegetables, and legumes. These foods are also high in fiber, which can help slow down glucose absorption into the bloodstream and promote feelings of fullness.

It's important to note that not all carbohydrates are created equal, and the carbohydrate source's quality can significantly impact blood sugar regulation. For example, whole fruits contain natural sugars. Still, they also contain fiber, vitamins, and minerals, making them a healthier option than fruit juice, which has a concentrated amount of sugar without the beneficial fiber.

The number of carbohydrates we consume can also impact blood sugar regulation. Consuming large amounts of carbohydrates at once can overwhelm the body's ability to produce enough insulin to regulate blood glucose levels properly. This can lead to hyperglycemia, characterized by high blood glucose levels, and can increase the risk of developing diabetes and other chronic health conditions.

To maintain healthy blood sugar levels, choosing complex carbohydrates and consuming them in moderation is essential. This can help to prevent blood sugar spikes and crashes, promote sustained energy levels, and reduce the risk of chronic health conditions associated with high blood sugar levels.

This page was left blank intentionally

Smart Carbs: Fuel Your Body and Shed Weight

Carbohydrates are one of our diet's three main macronutrients, protein and fat. They are our bodies' primary energy source and play a crucial role in maintaining blood sugar levels. However, not all carbs are created equal. Some carbs are quickly digested and cause a rapid spike in blood sugar levels, while others are digested slowly and provide a sustained release of energy.

Choosing the right carbs is essential for maintaining healthy blood sugar levels and promoting weight loss. Here are some tips for selecting smart carbs:

Choose complex carbs over simple carbs: Complex carbs, such as whole grains, fruits, and vegetables, are high in fiber and take longer to digest than simple carbs, such as candy and sugary drinks. This means they provide a steady stream of energy and keep you feeling full for longer.

Look for low glycemic index foods: The glycemic index (GI) measures how quickly a food raises blood sugar levels. Foods with a high GI cause a rapid spike in blood sugar levels, while foods with a low GI provide a slow, steady release of energy. Examples of low-GI foods include sweet potatoes, beans, and whole-grain bread.

Avoid refined carbs: Refined carbs, such as white bread and pasta, have been stripped of fiber and nutrients, leaving only the starchy endosperm. This makes them quickly digested and can cause a spike in blood sugar levels. Instead, opt for whole-grain versions of these fiber-rich foods that provide sustained energy.

Remember about fruit: Although fruit contains natural sugars, it is also high in fiber and nutrients. The fiber in fruit helps slow down the absorption of sugar into the bloodstream, making it a smart choice for maintaining healthy blood sugar levels.

By choosing smart carbs, you can fuel your body with the energy it needs while promoting weight loss and maintaining healthy blood sugar levels. Incorporate a variety of complex carbs into your diet, such as whole grains, fruits, and vegetables, and limit your intake of refined carbs and sugary foods. With a little effort and planning, you can make intelligent carb choices that will benefit your health in the long run.

The Science Behind Blood Sugar

Blood sugar and insulin

Blood sugar and insulin are intimately connected. Insulin is a hormone the pancreas produces that helps regulate blood sugar levels. It does this by allowing glucose, the sugar in the bloodstream, to be absorbed by the body's cells to be used for energy.

When we eat carbohydrates, they are broken down into glucose and enter the bloodstream. This triggers the pancreas to release insulin to help move glucose from the bloodstream into the cells. If too much glucose is in the bloodstream, the pancreas releases more insulin to bring blood sugar levels back down.

Insulin resistance occurs when the body's cells become less responsive to insulin. This means that more insulin is needed to get glucose into the cells, which can lead to high insulin levels in the bloodstream. This can eventually lead to prediabetes or type 2 diabetes.

High blood sugar levels over time can also damage organs and tissues in the body, leading to complications such as heart disease, nerve damage, kidney disease, and blindness.

Maintaining a healthy diet and lifestyle can help prevent insulin resistance and maintain healthy blood sugar levels. This includes consuming a balanced diet low in refined sugars and carbohydrates, regular exercise, managing stress levels, and getting enough sleep.

Additionally, it's essential to regularly monitor blood sugar levels, especially if you have risk factors for diabetes, such as being overweight, having a family history of diabetes, or having high blood pressure.

If you are concerned about your blood sugar levels or have a family history of diabetes, you must talk to your healthcare provider. They can help you understand your risks and guide you in maintaining healthy blood sugar levels.

Mastering the Balancing Act: How Your Body Regulates Blood Sugar

Blood sugar regulation is essential for maintaining good health. Our bodies rely on glucose, a type of sugar, as a primary energy source. However, too much or too little glucose in the bloodstream can have serious consequences. That's why the body has a sophisticated system to keep blood sugar levels within a narrow range. This book will explore how the body regulates blood sugar levels and why it's so important.

Glucose comes from the food we eat, mainly carbohydrates. When we eat a meal containing carbohydrates, our digestive system breaks them down into glucose and other sugars, which are absorbed into the bloodstream. As glucose concentration in the bloodstream increases, the pancreas releases a hormone called insulin into the bloodstream. Insulin's primary job is to help transport glucose from the bloodstream into the cells, which can be used as energy or stored for later use.

Insulin is a key that unlocks the cells' doors, allowing glucose to enter. Once inside, glucose is used immediately to fuel the cells' activities or stored in the liver and muscles as glycogen for later use. This process helps reduce the glucose concentration in the bloodstream, bringing it back to a more normal level.

When blood sugar levels drop too low, the body triggers a series of mechanisms to raise them. The pancreas releases a hormone called glucagon, which signals the liver to convert stored glycogen into glucose and release it into the bloodstream. This process, called glycogenolysis, helps raise blood sugar levels.

Another hormone that plays a role in blood sugar regulation is called cortisol. The adrenal glands produce cortisol in response to stress. It raises blood sugar levels by triggering the release of glucose from the liver.

In addition to insulin, glucagon, and cortisol, many other hormones and signaling molecules are involved in blood sugar regulation. For example, a hormone called amylin is produced by the pancreas along with insulin. Amylin slows down the rate at which glucose enters the bloodstream after a meal, helping to prevent spikes in blood sugar levels.

Various factors can influence the body's ability to regulate blood sugar levels. For example, certain medications can interfere with insulin's ability to transport glucose into cells. Stress can also raise blood sugar levels by increasing the production of cortisol. Lack of sleep, illness, and physical activity can also affect blood sugar regulation.

This page was left blank intentionally

Blood Sugar Demystified: Understanding Normal Levels and Diabetes

Blood sugar, or glucose, is a crucial component of our body. It provides the energy our cells need to function, allowing us to perform daily tasks and activities. However, when our blood sugar levels are not typical, it can lead to serious health complications, including diabetes.

This book will demystify blood sugar and help you understand normal levels and diabetes.

What are Normal Blood Sugar Levels?

Normal blood sugar levels are crucial to maintaining good health. Blood sugar levels can vary depending on various factors such as food intake, physical activity, and time of day. However, the American Diabetes Association (ADA) provides the following guidelines for normal blood sugar levels:

- Fasting blood sugar levels: Between 70-99 mg/dL
- Blood sugar levels before meals: 80-130 mg/dL

- Blood sugar levels after meals: Below 180 mg/dL

- It is important to note that these guidelines may vary depending on individual circumstances and health conditions.

What is Diabetes?

Diabetes is a chronic health condition that affects how your body processes blood sugar. The pancreas, an organ located in the abdomen, produces a hormone called insulin that regulates blood sugar levels. When you have diabetes, your body either doesn't produce enough insulin or cannot use it effectively, leading to high blood sugar levels.

There are two main types of diabetes:

Type 1 diabetes occurs when the body's immune system attacks and destroys the cells that produce insulin in the pancreas. Type 1 diabetes is typically diagnosed in childhood or adolescence and requires lifelong insulin therapy.

Type 2 diabetes occurs when the body becomes resistant to insulin or doesn't produce enough of it. Type 2 diabetes is more common and can be managed through lifestyle changes, medication, and insulin therapy.

What Causes Diabetes?

Several factors can contribute to the development of diabetes, including:

Genetics: If you have a family history of diabetes, you may be at a higher risk of developing the condition.

Obesity: Being overweight or obese can increase your risk of developing type 2 diabetes.

Physical inactivity: Lack of physical activity can lead to weight gain and increase your risk of developing diabetes.

Age: As you age, your risk of developing type 2 diabetes increases.

Gestational diabetes: This type of diabetes occurs during pregnancy and can increase your risk of developing type 2 diabetes later in life.

SYMPTOMS OF DIABETES

The symptoms of diabetes can vary depending on the type of diabetes and the severity of the condition. Some common symptoms of diabetes include:

- Frequent urination
- Excessive thirst
- Hunger
- Fatigue
- Blurred vision
- Slow-healing wounds
- Numbness or tingling in the hands or feet
- Weight loss (Type 1 diabetes)
- The increased appetite (Type 2 diabetes)

How to Manage Blood Sugar Levels

Managing blood sugar levels is essential for individuals with diabetes to avoid complications. Some effective strategies for controlling blood sugar levels include:

Following a healthy diet: Eating a well-balanced diet rich in whole grains, fruits, vegetables, and lean protein can help regulate blood sugar levels.

Physical activity: Regular exercise can help control blood sugar levels and improve insulin sensitivity.

Medication: Some people with diabetes may require a prescription to help manage blood sugar levels.

Blood sugar monitoring: Checking blood sugar levels regularly can help individuals with diabetes adjust their treatment plan accordingly.

This page was left blank intentionally

Balancing Blood Sugar with Protein and Healthy Fats

The Power Duo: Protein and Healthy Fats in Blood Sugar Control

Regarding blood sugar control, carbohydrates are often the first macronutrient that comes to mind. While it's true that carbs play a significant role in regulating blood sugar levels, protein, and healthy fats are equally important. This book will explore the power duo of protein and healthy fats and how they can help you maintain balanced blood sugar levels.

Protein and Blood Sugar:

Protein is an essential macronutrient that is crucial for a healthy diet. It plays a vital role in building and repairing tissues and providing energy to the body. But did you know protein also plays a role in blood sugar control? Consuming protein stimulates the release of a hormone called glucagon, which signals the liver to release stored glucose into the bloodstream. This helps to prevent blood sugar levels from dropping too low.

In addition, protein can help slow down carbohydrate absorption in the body. When we eat carbohydrates alone, they are rapidly digested and absorbed, leading to a quick spike in blood sugar levels. But when we combine carbohydrates with protein, carbs' digestion, and absorption are slowed, resulting in a more gradual and steady rise in blood sugar levels.

Healthy Fats and Blood Sugar:

Healthy fats are another vital macronutrient that can help to regulate blood sugar levels. When we consume healthy fats, such as those found in nuts, seeds, avocados, and fatty fish, they help to slow down the absorption of carbohydrates in the body. This results in a slower and more gradual rise in blood sugar levels.

In addition, healthy fats can help to increase insulin sensitivity in the body. Insulin is the hormone responsible for regulating blood sugar levels. When we become insulin resistant, our bodies can no longer effectively use insulin to regulate blood sugar levels. But consuming healthy fats can help improve insulin sensitivity, making it easier for our bodies to regulate blood sugar levels.

Tips for Incorporating Protein and Healthy Fats:

Now that you understand the role of protein and healthy fats in blood sugar regulation, here are some tips for incorporating them into your diet:

- Choose lean protein sources, such as chicken, fish, and tofu, and pair them with complex carbohydrates like quinoa, sweet potatoes, and brown rice.
- Incorporate healthy fats into your meals by adding avocado to your salad or using olive oil for cooking.
- Snack on nuts and seeds, such as almonds, walnuts, and pumpkin seeds, for a healthy dose of protein and healthy fats.

This page was left blank intentionally

Fueling Your Body Right: Smart Choices for Protein and Fat Sources

Protein, and healthy fats are just as essential as carbohydrates when maintaining healthy blood sugar levels. But not all protein and fat sources are created equal. This book will discuss the benefits of choosing suitable protein and fat sources for optimal blood sugar control and overall health.

Protein

Protein is an essential macronutrient in building and repairing tissues, producing enzymes and hormones, and maintaining a healthy immune system. It is also critical for stabilizing blood sugar levels by slowing glucose absorption into the bloodstream.

However, not all protein sources are created equal. Processed meats such as sausages, hot dogs, and deli meats are high in sodium and preservatives and are linked to an increased risk of diabetes and other health problems. Instead, opt for lean protein sources such as chicken, turkey, fish, beans, lentils, and tofu.

Fish is a perfect choice, as it is high in omega-3 fatty acids, which have been shown to improve insulin sensitivity and reduce inflammation. Aim for two servings of fish per week, choosing varieties such as salmon, mackerel, and sardines.

Avoid frying and grilling, baking, or roasting when preparing your protein sources. These methods will help retain your food's nutrients without adding excess fat and calories.

Healthy Fats

Healthy fats are essential to a balanced diet, providing energy, aiding in nutrient absorption, and promoting satiety. They are also crucial for regulating blood sugar levels by slowing glucose absorption into the bloodstream.

However, not all fats are created equal. Trans fats and saturated fats should be avoided, as they have been linked to an increased risk of heart disease and other health problems. Instead, use unsaturated fats such as olive oil, avocado, nuts, and seeds.

Nuts and seeds are excellent choices, as they are high in fiber and protein and have been shown to improve blood sugar control. They also make a great snack option when you're on the go. Just be mindful of portion sizes, as they are high in calories.

Avoid using vegetable oils such as canola and sunflower oil when cooking with fats, as they can be high in omega-6 fatty acids, which can contribute to inflammation. Instead, opt for olive or coconut oil, high in healthy monounsaturated and medium-chain triglyceride (MCT) fats, respectively.

This page was left blank intentionally

The Secret to Sustained Weight Loss and Health: A Balanced Diet

A balanced diet is essential for maintaining a healthy weight and overall well-being. While many diets focus on eliminating certain foods or food groups, a balanced diet is all about moderation and ensuring you're getting various nutrients. In this book, we'll explore the benefits of a balanced diet for sustained weight loss and health and tips for incorporating healthy foods into your diet.

What is a balanced diet?

A balanced diet includes a mix of carbohydrates, proteins, fats, vitamins, and minerals. The exact proportions may vary depending on your individual needs, but in general, a balanced diet should consist of the following:

- 45-65% of calories from carbohydrates, such as whole grains, fruits, and vegetables
- 10-35% of calories from protein, such as lean meats, fish, beans, and nuts
- 20-35% of calories from healthy fats, such as olive oil, avocados, and nuts

In addition to these macronutrients, a balanced diet should also include a variety of vitamins and minerals, such as vitamin D, calcium, and iron. These can be found in various foods, such as dairy products, leafy greens, and lean meats.

Benefits of a balanced diet:

Sustained weight loss: A balanced diet can help you lose and keep weight off. By incorporating a variety of nutrient-rich foods into your meals, you'll be less likely to feel deprived or hungry, which can lead to overeating or snacking on unhealthy foods.

Improved overall health: A balanced diet can help lower your risk of chronic diseases such as heart disease, diabetes, and some forms of cancer. By including various fruits, vegetables, whole grains, and lean proteins, you'll get the nutrients your body needs to function at its best.

Increased energy: Eating a balanced diet can help boost your energy levels, making staying active and productive throughout the day easier. Carbohydrates provide your body with the energy needed to function, while protein helps repair and build muscle, and healthy fats keep you full and satisfied.

Tips for incorporating healthy foods into your diet:

Focus on whole, nutrient-dense foods: Instead of processed foods or snacks, including more whole foods such as fruits, vegetables, whole grains, and lean proteins. These foods are typically more filling and satisfying than processed foods, which can help you eat less overall.

Experiment with new recipes: Trying new recipes can be fun to incorporate more healthy foods into your diet. Look for recipes that feature fresh, whole ingredients and experiment with different flavor combinations to keep things interesting.

Make healthy swaps: Small changes to your diet, such as swapping out refined carbohydrates for whole grains or choosing low-fat dairy products instead of full-fat, can help you cut calories and improve the nutritional content of your meals.

Plan: Planning your meals and snacks ahead of time can help you make healthier choices throughout the day. Try prepping meals or snacks on the weekends to have healthy options during the week.

A balanced diet is essential for sustained weight loss and overall health. Incorporating various nutrient-dense foods into your diet and focusing on moderation can improve your energy levels, lower your risk of chronic diseases, and maintain a healthy weight. Remember to experiment with new recipes, make healthy swaps, and plan to set yourself up for success.

Building a Balanced Plate

Bite-sized Success: The Power of Portion Control for Blood Sugar Control

Regarding regulating blood sugar levels, portion control is often overlooked. Overeating food, even healthy ones, can lead to spikes in blood sugar levels, negatively impacting overall health. This book will explore the importance of portion control for blood sugar regulation and provide practical tips for achieving a balanced diet.

The Basics of Portion Control:

Portion control refers to eating the appropriate amount for your body's needs. While everyone's caloric needs may vary based on age, gender, and activity level, portion control is a fundamental principle that applies to all.

The easiest way to ensure proper portion control is to use visual cues, such as the size of your hand or a deck of cards, to estimate serving sizes. For example, a serving of protein (such as chicken or fish) should be about the size of your palm, while a serving of vegetables should be about the size of your fist.

Another helpful tool for portion control is using smaller plates and bowls. Studies have shown that using smaller containers can lead to a decrease in calorie intake and an increase in satiety or feeling total.

Portion Control and Blood Sugar Regulation:

Regarding blood sugar regulation, portion control is essential for several reasons. First, overeating food, regardless of its nutritional value, can cause blood sugar levels to spike. This is because the body needs insulin to transport glucose (sugar) from the bloodstream to the cells for energy. Too much food can overwhelm the body's insulin response, leading to high blood sugar levels.

Additionally, portion control is essential for maintaining a balanced diet that includes a variety of foods. Consuming too much of any one type of food, even if it is healthy, can lead to imbalances in nutrient intake and potentially adverse health effects.

Practical Tips for Portion Control:

Now that we understand the importance of portion control for blood sugar regulation let's explore some practical tips for achieving a balanced diet.

Use visual cues: As mentioned earlier, visual cues such as the size of your hand or a deck of cards can help estimate serving sizes.

Fill up on non-starchy vegetables: Vegetables are an excellent source of fiber, vitamins, and minerals, and they are low in calories. Fill half of your plate with non-starchy vegetables such as broccoli, spinach, and peppers.

Practice mindful eating: Mindful eating involves paying attention to your food, chewing slowly, and savoring each bite. This can help you tune in to your body's hunger and fullness cues, leading to more appropriate portions.

Use smaller plates and bowls: As mentioned earlier, using smaller plates and bowls can help with portion control by tricking your brain into thinking you are eating more food than you are.

Don't skip meals: Skipping meals can lead to overeating later in the day and can cause blood sugar levels to spike. Aim to eat regular, balanced meals and snacks throughout the day.

Portion control is a simple yet powerful tool for achieving a balanced diet and regulating blood sugar levels. By using visual cues, filling up on non-starchy vegetables, practicing mindful eating, using smaller plates, and eating regular meals and snacks, you can maintain a healthy weight and reduce the risk of chronic diseases associated with high blood sugar levels.

Plate Power: Building a Balanced Meal for Lasting Energy and Weight Loss

When it comes to healthy eating, building a balanced plate is the key to success. A balanced meal can provide the nutrients your body needs to function correctly and help you achieve your weight loss goals. But what exactly does a balanced meal look like, and how can you ensure you get the proper nutrients in the right amounts?

A balanced meal is centered around including various food groups in appropriate proportions. These food groups include protein, carbohydrates, healthy fats, and vegetables. Here's how to build a balanced plate that can help you maintain steady energy levels and reach your weight loss goals:

Start with protein: Protein is an essential nutrient that helps build and repair tissues in the body. It also enables you to feel full for more extended periods. Aim for a serving of protein about the size of your palm. Good protein sources include chicken, turkey, fish, eggs, tofu, and legumes.

Add complex carbohydrates: Carbohydrates are a great energy source for the body, but not all carbohydrates are created equal. Focus on complex carbohydrates like whole grains, fruits, and vegetables rich in fiber, essential vitamins, and minerals. Aim for a serving of carbohydrates about the size of your fist.

Include healthy fats: Healthy fats, like those found in avocados, nuts, and olive oil, are essential for proper brain function and hormone production. They also help you feel full and satisfied after a meal. Aim for a serving of healthy fats that's about the size of your thumb.

Load up on vegetables: Vegetables are low in calories and fiber, so they can help you feel full without overloading on calories. They're also packed with essential vitamins and minerals for overall health. Aim to fill at least half of your plate with vegetables.

Remember portion sizes: Even if you're eating a balanced meal, portion sizes are still significant. Aim to keep your portion sizes in check by using smaller plates, measuring your food, and avoiding mindless snacking.

In addition to building a balanced plate, some other tips can help you maintain steady blood sugar levels and achieve weight loss goals. These include:

- Eating smaller, more frequent meals throughout the day instead of three large meals
- Drinking plenty of water to stay hydrated
- Avoiding sugary drinks and processed foods
- Eating slowly and mindfully helps you feel more satisfied

Following these tips and building a balanced plate can give your body the nutrients it needs to function correctly, maintain steady energy levels throughout the day, and achieve weight loss goals. Remember, healthy eating is all about balance and moderation, so don't be too hard on yourself if you slip up occasionally.

This page was left blank intentionally

Tips for meal planning and prepping

Meal planning and prepping are essential to maintaining a healthy diet and lifestyle. Planning and preparing meals in advance can save time and money and reduce the stress of mealtime decisions. This book will provide tips and tricks for successful meal planning and prepping.

Start with a plan

The first step in meal planning and prepping is to create a plan. Take some time each week to plan out your meals and snacks. This will help you stay organized and avoid last-minute decisions leading to unhealthy choices.

Start by deciding the number of meals and snacks you need for the week. Consider your schedule, events or commitments, and the number of people you feed. Then, plan out what you will eat for each meal and snack.

Make a grocery list

Once you have your meal plan, create a grocery list of all the necessary ingredients. This will help you stay on track when you go to the grocery store and prevent you from buying unnecessary items.

When making your list, include healthy options such as fruits, vegetables, lean proteins, and whole grains. Try to avoid processed and packaged foods as much as possible.

Prep ingredients in advance

Prepping ingredients in advance can save you time and make cooking meals easier. You can wash and chop vegetables, cook proteins, and prepare grains in advance. This will make assembling meals quick and easy.

Consider prepping ingredients on a designated day of the week, such as Sunday, when you have more free time. You can also prepare meals for the week and store them in the fridge or freezer.

Use meal prep containers.

Investing in suitable quality meal prep containers can make meal planning and prep more efficient. These containers are designed to keep food fresh and easily stored in the fridge or freezer.

Choose containers that are microwave-safe and easy to clean. You can find them in various sizes and shapes to accommodate different types of food.

Cook in bulk

Cooking in bulk can save you time and money. You can make large batches of soups, stews, casseroles, and other dishes and freeze them for later.

Consider using a slow or pressure cooker to make large batches of meals with minimal effort. These appliances can cook food while you're away, bringing you home to a hot, nutritious meal.

Keep healthy snacks on hand.

Healthy snacks can prevent you from reaching for unhealthy options when hunger strikes. Keep snacks such as fruit, nuts, and cut-up vegetables readily available.

Consider portioning snacks in advance using small bags or containers. This can help prevent overeating and make it easier to grab a snack on the go.

Don't be afraid to try new things.

Meal planning and prepping can be great opportunities to try new foods and recipes. Experiment with different cuisines, ingredients, and cooking techniques.

You can find inspiration for new recipes online, in cookbooks, or by asking friends and family for their favorite recipes. Don't be afraid to get creative and have fun with your meal planning and prepping.

In conclusion, meal planning and prepping can help you save time and money and make healthier choices. Following these tips, you can successfully plan and prepare nutritious meals for yourself and your family. Remember to stay flexible and have fun with your meal planning and prepping.

This page was left blank intentionally

Smart Snacking for Balanced Blood Sugar

Snacks in blood sugar regulation

Snacking is an integral part of our daily food intake. It keeps us energized, helps prevent overeating at mealtime, and can even improve our metabolism. However, for people with blood sugar issues, snacking can be a challenge. The wrong snack can cause a spike in blood sugar levels, leading to a crash later.

But with the right choices, snacking can help regulate blood sugar levels and keep us feeling full and satisfied. In this book, we will explore the role of snacks in blood sugar regulation and provide tips for making wise choices.

Understanding Blood Sugar Regulation

Before diving into snacks' role in blood sugar regulation, let's first review how the body regulates blood sugar. When we eat carbohydrates, they are broken down into glucose, which enters the bloodstream. The pancreas then releases insulin, which allows glucose to enter the cells and be used for energy. When blood sugar levels drop, the pancreas releases glucagon, which prompts the liver to release stored glucose into the bloodstream. This balance between insulin and glucagon helps maintain stable blood sugar levels.

However, for people with blood sugar issues such as diabetes, this system can be disrupted. In type 1 diabetes, the body does not produce enough insulin, while in type 2 diabetes, the body becomes resistant to insulin. This can cause blood sugar levels to become too high or too low, leading to various health problems.

Snacks and Blood Sugar Regulation

Snacks can be a great way to keep blood sugar levels stable throughout the day. When we go long periods without eating, our blood sugar levels can drop, causing us to feel hungry and sluggish. Eating a healthy snack can help prevent this drop and keep us feeling energized.

However, not all snacks are created equal. Some snacks can cause blood sugar levels to spike, leading to a crash later on. The key is to choose snacks that are low in sugar and high in fiber and protein. This will help slow glucose absorption into the bloodstream, preventing a sudden spike in blood sugar levels.

Smart Snack Choices

So, what are some intelligent snack choices for blood sugar regulation? Here are some ideas:

Nuts: Nuts are a great source of healthy fats, protein, and fiber. They are also low in carbohydrates, making them an excellent snack for people with blood sugar issues. Choose unsalted varieties to avoid excess sodium.

Greek yogurt: Greek yogurt is high in protein and low in sugar, making it an ideal snack for blood sugar regulation. Add some berries or nuts for added fiber and flavor.

Hummus and veggies: Hummus is made from chickpeas, a good protein and fiber source. Pair it with raw veggies like carrots or celery for a low-carbohydrate snack.

Hard-boiled eggs: Hard-boiled eggs are a great source of protein and healthy fats. They are also low in carbohydrates, making them a smart snack for blood sugar regulation.

Cheese and apple slices: Pairing cheese with apple slices is a great way to balance protein, fiber, and carbohydrates. Choose a low-fat cheese to keep the calorie count in check.

Roasted chickpeas: Roasted chickpeas are a crunchy, high-protein snack that can help keep you feeling full and satisfied. Please make your own by tossing chickpeas with olive oil and your favorite spices, then roasting them in the oven.

Snack Smart: Healthy Snack Choices for Steady Blood Sugar

Snacking is an essential aspect of our daily lives. We all have cravings for something sweet or savory between meals. But when it comes to blood sugar regulation, choosing the right snacks can make a big difference. Consuming snacks high in sugar or refined carbohydrates can cause a rapid spike in blood sugar levels, leading to a crash in energy levels later. This book will discuss some healthy snack options that won't spike blood sugar levels and keep you energized throughout the day.

Nuts:

Nuts are a great snack option for people with diabetes as they are low in carbohydrates and high in healthy fats, fiber, and protein. They are also rich in nutrients like magnesium and vitamin E, essential for blood sugar regulation. A handful of nuts like almonds, cashews, or walnuts can provide a quick energy boost and keep you full for extended periods.

Seeds:

Seeds like chia, flax, and pumpkin seeds are excellent snack options for people with diabetes as they are low in carbohydrates, fiber, and healthy fats. They are also a good source of essential minerals like magnesium and zinc, which are necessary for blood sugar regulation. Add them to your yogurt, smoothies, or salads for an extra crunch.

Greek Yogurt:

Greek yogurt is a protein-rich snack option that can help stabilize blood sugar levels. It is low in carbohydrates and high in calcium and vitamin D, which are essential for bone health. You can add some fresh berries or nuts to your Greek yogurt for a tasty and nutritious snack.

Hard-boiled Eggs:

Hard-boiled eggs are a good source of protein, which can help stabilize blood sugar levels. They are also low in carbohydrates and high in essential nutrients like vitamin D and choline. You can sprinkle salt and pepper or add sliced avocado for a tasty and nutritious snack.

Vegetables with Hummus:

Vegetables like carrots, cucumbers, and bell peppers are low in carbohydrates and high in fiber and essential vitamins and minerals. Pairing them with hummus, which is made from chickpeas, can add some protein and healthy fats to your snack. Hummus is also a good source of fiber, which can help regulate blood sugar levels.

Cheese:

Cheese is a protein-rich snack option that can help stabilize blood sugar levels. It is also low in carbohydrates and high in calcium and vitamin D, which are essential for bone health. You can pair some cheese with crackers or sliced vegetables for a tasty and nutritious snack.

Avocado:

Avocado is a healthy, fat-rich snack that can help stabilize blood sugar levels. It is also low in carbohydrates and high in fiber and essential vitamins and minerals like vitamin C and potassium. You can mash some avocado on a slice of whole-grain toast or add it to your salad for a nutritious snack.

Choosing healthy snacks that won't spike blood sugar levels is essential for people with diabetes. Snacks that are low in carbohydrates and high in fiber, healthy fats, and protein can help stabilize blood sugar levels and provide a sustained energy boost. Incorporating snacks like nuts, seeds, Greek yogurt, hard-boiled eggs, and vegetables with hummus, cheese, and avocado can help you maintain a balanced and healthy diet.

Tips for snacking on the go and at home

Snacking can be a great way to curb hunger and maintain energy levels throughout the day. However, making healthy snack choices is essential that won't negatively impact your blood sugar levels. In this book, we'll discuss some tips for snacking on the go and at home to keep your blood sugar in check.

Plan Ahead

The key to healthy snacking is planning. Take some time to think about your snacks for the day or week and prepare them in advance. This can help you avoid reaching for unhealthy options when hunger strikes. Some great snack ideas include cut-up veggies, fresh fruit, hard-boiled eggs, unsweetened Greek yogurt, and nuts.

Read Labels

When selecting pre-packaged snacks, it's essential to read labels carefully. Many packaged snacks can be high in sugar and refined carbohydrates, which can cause blood sugar levels to spike. Look for snacks that are low in sugar and high in fiber and protein. Aim for snacks with less than 10 grams of sugar per serving.

Portion Control

Even healthy snacks can lead to overeating if you're not careful. It's important to practice portion control when snacking. Measure out your snacks in advance to avoid mindlessly eating a bag of nuts or a whole container of hummus. Pre-portioned snack packs are also a great option.

Choose Whole Foods

Whole foods, such as fruits, vegetables, and nuts, are the best choices for snacking. They are nutrient-dense and balance carbohydrates, protein, and healthy fats well. Avoid processed snacks, such as chips and candy, as they are often high in calories, sugar, and unhealthy fats.

Don't Skip Meals

While snacking can be a great way to curb hunger, it's important not to rely on snacks as a meal substitute.

Skipping meals can cause blood sugar levels to drop too low, leading to cravings and overeating later. Make sure to include a variety of healthy foods in your meals to keep your blood sugar levels stable throughout the day.

Pack Snacks for the Road

When you're on the go, grabbing a quick and unhealthy snack can be tempting. However, with some planning, you can pack healthy snacks to take with you on the road. Some great options include fruit, trail mix, protein bars, and cut-up veggies. Packing snacks can help you save money and avoid unhealthy fast-food options.

Experiment with Flavor

Healthy snacking doesn't have to be boring. Experiment with different flavors and spices to make your snacks more exciting. Add cinnamon to your yogurt or apple slices, or sprinkle paprika on your roasted chickpeas. Healthy snacks can be just as delicious as unhealthy ones.

In conclusion, snacking can be a great way to maintain energy levels throughout the day. However, making healthy snack choices is essential to keep your blood sugar levels stable. By planning, reading labels, practicing portion control, choosing whole foods, not skipping meals, packing snacks for the road, and experimenting with flavor, you can enjoy healthy and delicious snacks that won't negatively impact your blood sugar levels.

Burn and Balance: The Role of Exercise in Blood Sugar Control

Burn Fat, Not Sugar

Exercise is often touted as an essential component of a healthy lifestyle, and for a good reason. Not only can it help with weight loss and muscle gain, but it can also play a significant role in blood sugar regulation. In this book, we'll take a closer look at the effect of exercise on blood sugar levels, the types of exercise that are most effective for blood sugar control, and the benefits of exercise for overall health and well-being.

How does exercise affect blood sugar?

When you exercise, your body uses glucose as fuel for your muscles. As a result, your muscles become more sensitive to insulin, the hormone that helps regulate blood sugar levels. This increased sensitivity means that your muscles can better absorb glucose from your bloodstream, which can help lower blood sugar levels.

Additionally, exercise can help to reduce insulin resistance, which is a condition that occurs when your body becomes less responsive to insulin over time. Insulin resistance is a hallmark of type 2 diabetes, and it can lead to chronically elevated blood sugar levels if left unchecked. Regular exercise can help to reverse insulin resistance and improve your body's ability to regulate blood sugar.

What types of exercise are best for blood sugar control?

Any exercise can help to improve blood sugar regulation, but some types may be more effective than others. Aerobic activities like brisk walking, cycling, or swimming are considered the most effective for controlling blood sugar. This is because aerobic exercise engages large muscle groups and requires a sustained level of activity, which helps to maximize glucose uptake by the muscles.

Resistance training, such as weightlifting or bodyweight exercises, can also be practical for blood sugar control. This is because resistance training helps build muscle mass, improving insulin sensitivity and glucose uptake in the muscles.

Finally, high-intensity interval training (HIIT) efficiently regulates blood sugar. HIIT involves short bursts of intense exercise followed by periods of rest or low-intensity exercise. This type of training has been shown to improve insulin sensitivity and glucose uptake in the muscles, and it may also help to increase overall fitness and metabolic health.

What are the benefits of exercise for blood sugar control?

In addition to improving blood sugar regulation, regular exercise has numerous other benefits for overall health and well-being. These include:

Weight loss: Exercise can help to promote weight loss by burning calories and increasing metabolism. This can be especially important for people with type 2 diabetes, as excess weight can contribute to insulin resistance and chronically elevated blood sugar levels.

Improved cardiovascular health: Regular exercise can help to lower blood pressure, reduce inflammation, and improve cholesterol levels, all of which can contribute to better cardiovascular health.

Reduced stress: Exercise has been shown to help reduce stress and improve mood, which can positively impact blood sugar regulation. Chronic stress has been linked to insulin resistance and elevated blood sugar levels, so finding ways to manage stress is essential for overall health.

Increased energy: Regular exercise can help to boost energy levels and reduce fatigue, which can be especially beneficial for people with diabetes who may experience fluctuations in energy levels throughout the day.

Improved overall health: Exercise has been shown to reduce the risk of numerous chronic diseases, including heart disease, stroke, and certain types of cancer. By improving overall health, regular exercise can help to reduce the risk of complications associated with diabetes.

In conclusion, an exercise is a powerful tool for blood sugar regulation and overall health. By engaging in regular aerobic exercise, resistance training, or HIIT, you can improve insulin sensitivity and glucose uptake in the muscles, helping to regulate blood sugar levels and reduce the risk of complications associated with diabetes.

Move More, Live Better: Easy Ways to Incorporate Physical Activity into Your Daily Routine

In today's sedentary lifestyle, finding the motivation to be physically active can be challenging. Many of us sit for hours at work or home, which can affect our overall health and well-being. However, incorporating physical activity into our daily routine can have numerous benefits, including improved blood sugar regulation, weight loss, and increased energy levels. This book will explore easy and practical ways to move more and live better.

Take the Stairs

Taking the stairs instead of the elevator is an easy way to incorporate physical activity into your daily routine. Climbing stairs burns calories and provides a cardiovascular workout, making it an excellent way to improve blood sugar regulation and overall health. If you work in a multi-story building, try taking the stairs instead of the elevator at least once daily and gradually increase the frequency as you become more comfortable.

Walk More

Walking is one of the most straightforward and accessible forms of physical activity. It is a low-impact exercise that can be done almost anywhere and requires no special equipment. Try incorporating more walking into your daily routine, whether during your lunch break or walking to nearby places instead of driving. Aim for at least 30 minutes of walking daily, gradually increasing the duration and intensity as you become more comfortable.

Stand More

Sitting for long periods can adversely affect our health, including poor blood sugar regulation and weight gain. Incorporating standing into your daily routine can help counteract the adverse effects of prolonged sitting. Consider standing during phone calls or meetings or investing in a standing desk for your workspace. Standing engages the muscles and burns more calories than sitting, making it an easy and practical way to move and live better.

Incorporate Strength Training

Strength training involves using resistance to build muscle and can have numerous benefits, including improved blood sugar regulation, weight loss, and increased metabolism. Incorporating strength training into your routine can be as simple as doing bodyweight exercises, such as push-ups and squats, or using resistance bands or weights. Aim to incorporate strength training exercises at least two to three times a week for optimal results.

Find an Activity You Enjoy

Physical activity does not have to be a chore. Finding an enjoyable activity can make it easier to incorporate into your daily routine and increase your motivation to be more physically active. Try different activities, such as dancing, swimming, or yoga, until you find one you enjoy. This can make sticking to a routine more accessible and improve overall health and well-being.

In conclusion, incorporating physical activity into your daily routine can have numerous benefits, including improved blood sugar regulation, weight loss, and increased energy levels. You can move and live better by taking the stairs, walking more, standing more, incorporating strength training, and finding an activity you enjoy. Start small and gradually increase your physical activity level to reap the full benefits of a more active lifestyle.

Breaking Through the Barriers: How to Stay Motivated for Fitness Success

Starting a fitness routine is easy, but staying motivated to continue can be challenging. Many physical activity barriers, such as lack of time, energy, or resources, can make staying committed to a fitness routine difficult. However, with helpful tips and strategies, you can overcome these barriers and stay motivated to achieve your fitness goals.

Set Realistic Goals

Setting realistic goals is an essential step in staying motivated. Be honest about what you can achieve, and make sure your goals are achievable. Setting unrealistic goals will only lead to frustration and disappointment. When setting goals, it is essential to be specific, measurable, attainable, relevant, and time-bound. For example, instead of saying, "I want to get fit," set a goal like "I want to walk for 30 minutes a day, five days a week, for the next month."

Find an Accountability Partner

Having an accountability partner can be a great way to stay motivated. You can work out together, share progress, and motivate each other. Choose someone who shares your fitness goals and is committed to achieving them. This person can be a friend, family member, or personal trainer.

Mix it Up

Doing the same workout every day can become monotonous and boring. Mixing your routine with different exercises can make it more exciting and challenging. Try a new workout class, incorporate strength training into your practice, or take up a new sport.

Create a Routine

Creating a routine can make physical activity a habit. Schedule your workout simultaneously every day so it becomes part of your daily routine. Set a reminder on your phone, or use a fitness app to keep you on track.

Reward Yourself

Rewarding yourself for reaching fitness goals can be a great way to stay motivated. Choose a reward that is meaningful to you, such as a massage or a new workout outfit. Celebrating your successes will help keep you motivated to continue working towards your fitness goals.

Overcome Excuses

Excuses are one of the most significant barriers to physical activity. If you make excuses, such as "I'm too tired" or "I don't have time," it's time to overcome them. Instead of saying, "I don't have time to work out," try saying, "I will make time to work out." Replace negative self-talk with positive affirmations to help overcome excuses.

Track Your Progress

Tracking your progress can be a great way to stay motivated. Use a fitness tracker or app to follow your steps, distance, and calories burned. Seeing progress can help motivate you and show you how far you've come.

Find Joy in Exercise

Physical activity doesn't have to be a chore. Find a type of exercise you enjoy, whether dancing, hiking, or swimming. Training should be fun, not a punishment. When you find joy in an activity, staying motivated is easier.

Get Enough Rest and Recovery

Rest and recovery are essential components of a successful fitness routine. Ensure you get enough rest and allow your body time to recover between workouts. Overtraining can lead to burnout and injury, making it harder to stay motivated.

Be Patient

Fitness is a journey, not a destination. It takes time to see results, so be patient with yourself. Keep going if you see immediate results. Remember that small changes can lead to significant progress over time.

Sleep and Stress Management

Snooze, Stress, and Sugar: The Surprising Connection You Need to Know

Sleep, stress, and blood sugar regulation are all interconnected. When we don't get enough sleep, we tend to feel more stressed, and our blood sugar levels can become imbalanced. On the other hand, when we are stressed, our rest can suffer, and our blood sugar can also be affected. This book will explore the link between sleep, stress, and blood sugar regulation and provide tips for improving each aspect of our health.

What is Blood Sugar Regulation?

Blood sugar regulation refers to the process of maintaining stable levels of glucose in the bloodstream. Glucose is the primary energy source for our bodies, and it comes from our foods. When we eat carbohydrates, they are broken down into glucose and released into the bloodstream. Insulin, a hormone produced by the pancreas, helps to transport glucose from the bloodstream into our cells, where it can be used for energy.

When our blood sugar levels are too high, it can lead to hyperglycemia, which can cause damage to our organs and blood vessels over time. When our blood sugar levels are too low, it can lead to hypoglycemia, which can cause symptoms such as dizziness, confusion, and even loss of consciousness.

Sleep and Blood Sugar Regulation

Getting enough sleep is essential for maintaining healthy blood sugar levels. When we don't get enough sleep, our bodies produce more stress hormone cortisol, which can cause our blood sugar levels to rise. In addition, lack of sleep can disrupt the balance of other hormones that regulate blood sugar, such as insulin and glucagon.

A study published in Diabetes Care found that people who slept less than six hours per night had higher fasting blood sugar levels and were more likely to develop type 2 diabetes than those who slept for seven to eight hours per night. Another study published in the journal sleep found that sleep deprivation can cause insulin resistance, a condition in which the body becomes less sensitive to the effects of insulin, leading to higher blood sugar levels.

TIPS FOR IMPROVING SLEEP

Stick to a regular sleep schedule: Go to bed and wake up simultaneously every day, even on weekends.

Create a sleep-friendly environment: Ensure your bedroom is dark, calm, and quiet, and avoid using electronic devices before bed.

Limit caffeine and alcohol: Caffeine and alcohol can interfere with sleep quality, so limiting your intake is best, especially before bedtime.

Relax before bed:
- Take a warm bath.
- Read a book.
- Practice relaxation techniques like deep breathing or meditation to help you wind down before bed.

Stress and Blood Sugar Regulation

Stress can also have a significant impact on blood sugar regulation. When we are under pressure, our bodies produce more cortisol and adrenaline, which can cause our blood sugar levels to rise. In addition, stress can lead to overeating or choosing unhealthy foods, which can also affect blood sugar levels.

A study published in the journal Psych neuroendocrinology found that chronic stress can cause insulin resistance, leading to higher blood sugar levels and an increased risk of type 2 diabetes. Another study published in Diabetes Care found that stress can lead to elevated blood sugar levels in people with type 2 diabetes.

TIPS FOR MANAGING STRESS

Exercise: Exercise is a great way to reduce stress and improve blood sugar regulation. Aim for at least 30 minutes of moderate-intensity exercise most days of the week.

Practice relaxation techniques: Deep breathing, meditation, yoga, and tai chi are all effective ways to reduce stress and improve blood sugar regulation.

Get social support:
- Talking to friends and family.
- Joining a support group.
- Seeing a therapist can help reduce stress levels and improve mental health.

Taking breaks throughout the day, whether a short walk or just a few minutes of deep breathing, can help reduce stress and improve productivity.

Get enough sleep: As mentioned earlier, getting enough sleep is crucial for managing stress levels.

Blood Sugar Regulation and Stress Management

In addition to improving sleep and managing stress, there are several other ways to maintain healthy blood sugar levels.

Eat a healthy diet: A balanced diet with plenty of fruits, vegetables, whole grains, and lean proteins can help regulate blood sugar levels. Avoid sugary or processed foods, which can cause blood sugar spikes.

Stay hydrated: Drinking plenty of water can help stabilize blood sugar levels.

Monitor blood sugar levels: If you have diabetes or are at risk for developing it, regularly monitoring your blood sugar levels can help you adjust your diet and lifestyle as needed.

Take medications as prescribed: If you have diabetes, taking medications as prescribed by your doctor is essential for managing blood sugar levels.

Sleep, stress, and blood sugar regulation are all closely linked. Getting enough sleep, managing stress, and maintaining a healthy lifestyle can all help regulate blood sugar levels and reduce the risk of developing diabetes. By incorporating the tips mentioned in this book, you can take steps toward improving your overall health and well-being. Remember, small changes can make a big difference over time, so start making positive changes today.

This page was left blank intentionally

How to be 10x better

Have you ever felt like you could be doing better in life? You may want to be more productive at work, have more energy for your hobbies, or feel better overall. The good news is that by improving your sleep quality and managing your stress levels, you can take significant steps towards becoming 10x better. Not only will you feel more energized and productive, but you will also improve your blood sugar control, reducing your risk of developing type 2 diabetes. This book will explore how you can improve your sleep quality and manage your stress levels for better blood sugar control and overall health.

Why is Sleep Important for Blood Sugar Control?

Getting enough high-quality sleep is crucial for maintaining healthy blood sugar levels. When we sleep, our bodies work to repair and restore themselves, including regulating glucose levels. If we don't get enough sleep or have poor sleep quality, it can lead to imbalanced blood sugar levels.

One study published in the Journal of Clinical Endocrinology and Metabolism found that people who slept for less than six hours per night had higher blood glucose levels and were more likely to develop insulin resistance than those who slept for seven to eight hours per night. Another study published in the Journal of Sleep Research found that poor sleep quality was associated with higher hemoglobin A1c (HbA1c) levels, a marker of long-term blood sugar control.

TIPS FOR IMPROVING SLEEP QUALITY

Stick to a sleep schedule: Try to go to bed and wake up simultaneously every day, even on weekends.

Create a sleep-conducive environment: Ensure your bedroom is calm, dark, and quiet. Avoid using electronic devices before bed, and consider investing in comfortable bedding.

Limit caffeine and alcohol: Both caffeine and alcohol can interfere with sleep quality. Limit your intake, especially in the hours leading up to bedtime.

Relax before bed:
- Take a warm bath.
- Read a book.

- Practice relaxation techniques like deep breathing or meditation to help you wind down before bed.

Exercise regularly: Regular exercise can help improve sleep quality. Aim for at least 30 minutes of moderate-intensity exercise most days of the week.

Why is Managing Stress Important for Blood Sugar Control?

Stress is a standard part of modern life, but chronic stress can hurt our health, including blood sugar control. When stressed, our bodies release cortisol, which raises blood sugar levels. Over time, this can lead to insulin resistance and an increased risk of type 2 diabetes.

One study published in the journal Psych neuroendocrinology found that people who experienced chronic stress had higher blood glucose levels and were more likely to develop type 2 diabetes. Another study published in Diabetes Care found that stress can cause blood sugar spikes in people with type 2 diabetes.

Tips for Managing Stress:

Practice relaxation techniques: Deep breathing, meditation, yoga, and tai chi are all effective ways to reduce stress and improve blood sugar control.

Regular exercise is a great way to reduce stress and improve blood sugar control. Aim for at least 30 minutes of moderate-intensity exercise most days of the week.

Prioritize self-care: Make time for activities you enjoy, whether reading, listening to music, or spending time with loved ones.

Get enough sleep: As mentioned earlier, high-quality sleep is crucial for managing stress levels.

Seek support:
- Talking to friends and family.
- Joining a support group.
- Seeing a therapist can help reduce stress levels and improve mental health.

Other Ways to Improve Blood Sugar Control:

Eating a healthy diet is crucial for maintaining healthy blood sugar levels. A balanced diet with plenty of fruits, vegetables, whole grains, and lean proteins can help regulate blood sugar levels. Avoid sugary or processed foods, which can cause blood sugar spikes.

Stay hydrated

Drinking plenty of water can help keep blood sugar levels stable. Aim for at least eight glasses of water daily, and more if you exercise or in a hot environment.

Monitor blood sugar levels.

If you have diabetes or are at risk for developing it, monitoring your blood sugar levels regularly can help you adjust your diet and lifestyle as needed. Your doctor can help determine how often you need to check your blood sugar levels.

Take medications as prescribed.

If you have diabetes, taking medications as your doctor prescribes is essential for managing blood sugar levels. Be sure to bring your medications on schedule and follow any dietary or lifestyle recommendations your healthcare provider provides.

By improving your sleep quality and managing your stress levels, you can take significant steps towards becoming 10x better. Not only will you feel more energized and productive, but you will also improve your blood sugar control, reducing your risk of developing type 2 diabetes. Incorporating the tips mentioned in this book, such as sticking to a sleep schedule, practicing relaxation techniques, eating a healthy diet, staying hydrated, and monitoring your blood sugar levels, can help you achieve better sleep and reduce stress and more nutritional blood sugar levels. Remember that small changes can make a big difference over time, so start making positive changes today.

Healthy Sleep Routine

Getting enough quality sleep is essential for our overall health and well-being. A healthy sleep routine can help us feel energized, productive, and mentally sharp throughout the day. This book will discuss some tips for creating a healthy sleep routine that works for you.

Stick to a consistent sleep schedule

A consistent sleep schedule is one of the most important aspects of a healthy sleep routine. This means going to bed and waking up simultaneously every day, even on weekends. When we stick to a consistent sleep schedule, our bodies learn to anticipate when it is time to sleep and wake up, which can help us fall asleep faster and feel refreshed.

Create a relaxing bedtime routine

Creating a relaxing bedtime routine can help signal our bodies that it is time to wind down and prepare for sleep. This could include taking a warm bath, reading a book, practicing yoga or meditation, or listening to calming music. Avoiding stimulating activities, such as watching TV or using electronic devices, before bedtime can also help promote relaxation.

Create a sleep-conducive environment

Creating a sleep-conducive environment is another essential aspect of a healthy sleep routine. This means ensuring that your bedroom is calm, dark, and quiet. Investing in a comfortable mattress and pillows can also help improve the quality of your sleep. Use earplugs or a white noise machine to block out unwanted sounds if noise is a problem.

Limit caffeine and alcohol consumption

Caffeine and alcohol consumption can both have a significant impact on our sleep quality. While caffeine can help us feel alert and awake during the day, consuming it later can interfere with our ability to fall asleep at night. Similarly, while alcohol can initially make us tired, it can also disrupt our sleep patterns, leading to poor-quality sleep.

Exercise regularly

Regular exercise can help promote better sleep by reducing stress and anxiety and promoting feelings of relaxation. Aim to get at least 30 minutes of moderate-intensity exercise most days of the week, but avoid exercising too close to bedtime, as this can interfere with your ability to fall asleep.

Avoid eating large meals before bedtime

Eating a large meal before bedtime can make it difficult to fall asleep and lead to indigestion and discomfort during the night. Instead, aim to eat your last meal of the day at least 2-3 hours before bedtime. If you need a snack before bed, choose something light and easy to digest, such as fruit or a small serving of yogurt.

Manage stress

Stress and anxiety can significantly impact our sleep quality, making it more difficult to fall and stay asleep. To manage stress, try incorporating relaxation techniques, such as deep breathing, meditation, or progressive muscle relaxation, into your bedtime routine. You may also want to consider speaking with a mental health professional if you are experiencing significant levels of stress or anxiety.

This page was left blank intentionally

Living with Balanced Blood Sugar for Lifelong Health

Balanced blood sugar levels are essential for lifelong health. The body relies on glucose, a type of sugar, as its primary energy source. However, when blood sugar levels become too high or too low, it can lead to various health problems, including diabetes, heart disease, and cognitive decline. This book will discuss how to live with balanced blood sugar for lifelong health.

Eat a balanced diet

Eating a balanced diet is one of the most important ways to maintain blood sugar levels. This means including nutrient-dense foods, such as whole grains, fruits and vegetables, lean protein, and healthy fats. It is also essential to avoid consuming too many processed foods and added sugars, as these can cause blood sugar levels to spike.

Stay hydrated

Drinking plenty of water is another essential aspect of maintaining balanced blood sugar levels. When dehydrated, our blood becomes thicker, making it more difficult for insulin to transport glucose into our cells. Aim to drink at least eight glasses of water daily and avoid sugary drinks, which can cause blood sugar levels to spike.

Exercise regularly

Regular exercise is essential for maintaining balanced blood sugar levels. Exercise helps our muscles use glucose more effectively, which can help prevent spikes in blood sugar levels. Aim to get at least 30 minutes of moderate-intensity exercise most days of the week, such as brisk walking, cycling, or swimming.

Manage stress

Stress can have a significant impact on our blood sugar levels. When we are stressed, our bodies release stress hormones, which can cause blood sugar levels to spike. Try incorporating relaxation techniques into your daily routine, such as deep breathing, meditation, or yoga, to manage stress. You may also want to consider speaking with a mental health professional if you are experiencing significant levels of stress or anxiety.

Get enough sleep

Getting enough quality sleep is essential for maintaining balanced blood sugar levels. When we are sleep deprived, our bodies become less sensitive to insulin, which can lead to spikes in blood sugar levels. Aim to get at least seven to eight hours of sleep per night and establish a consistent sleep schedule to help regulate your body's internal clock.

Monitor your blood sugar levels.

If you have a history of high blood sugar levels, monitoring your blood sugar levels regularly is essential. This can help you identify patterns and adjust your diet and lifestyle. Talk to your healthcare provider about how often you should check your blood sugar levels and your target range.

Take medication as prescribed.

If you have been diagnosed with diabetes, taking any medication prescribed by your healthcare provider as directed is essential. Drugs such as insulin can help regulate blood sugar levels and prevent complications associated with high blood sugar levels. Follow your healthcare provider's instructions carefully and report any side effects or concerns.

Maintaining balanced blood sugar levels is essential for lifelong health. By eating a balanced diet, staying hydrated, exercising regularly, managing stress, getting enough sleep, monitoring your blood sugar levels, and taking medication as prescribed, you can help prevent complications associated with high blood sugar levels and enjoy a healthy, fulfilling life. Remember to work closely with your healthcare provider to develop a personalized plan that works for you, and be sure to make any necessary adjustments as your needs change over time. You can live with balanced blood sugar and achieve lifelong health with the right approach.

Conclusion

In conclusion, outsmarting blood sugar is not about quick fixes or fad diets. It's about making sustainable lifestyle changes to prevent disease, promote weight loss, and improve overall health. By adopting healthy habits such as eating a balanced diet, staying hydrated, exercising regularly, managing stress, getting enough sleep, monitoring blood sugar levels, and taking medication as prescribed, we can take control of our health and live our best lives.

Remember that small changes can lead to significant results. Start by setting achievable goals and taking baby steps towards a healthier lifestyle. Celebrate your successes along the way, and don't be too hard on yourself if you slip up. Health is a journey, not a destination, and every step in the right direction is worth celebrating.

Finally, don't be afraid to seek support from friends, family, and healthcare professionals. It takes a village to outsmart blood sugar, and having a support system can make all the difference. Together, we can take control of our health and prevent disease, lose weight, and live healthier, happier lives. So let's get started and outsmart blood sugar, once and for all.

www.ingramcontent.com/pod-product-compliance
Lightning Source LLC
Chambersburg PA
CBHW061354250726
48657CB00004B/1481